# A Special Message from the Authors

Hello! Colin and I would like to thank you for loving yourself enough to begin or continue on a journey of great health and well-being. We see the greatness in you.

"Choose to be in Close Proximity to People who are empowering ... Who See the Greatness in You!" ~Wayne Dyer

Being lovers of food, we knew there was a more enjoyable way to prepare the limited foods on this protocol. Our prayer is that you enjoy this recipe book as much as we enjoyed making it.

God Bless and Namaste

*Colin and Jayne*

# PHASE II

## CONTENTS

# PHASE III

## CONTENTS

# HCG ESSENTIALS

- Meditation for Manifestation Download Dr. Wayne Dyer
- Food Scale
- Garlic & Pepper Grinder
- George Forman Grill
- Organic Extra Virgin Olive Oil
- Cooking Spray
- Oil Free Lotion
- Mineral Oil – Baby Oil
- Accurate Weight Scale
- Tape Measure
- Daily Weight Journal

## Seasonings

- Apple Cider Vinegar

- All Natural Liquid Aminos

- Stevia Natural Sweetener

- Sea Salt

- Paprika Ginger Root Black Pepper

- Cinnamon Parsley Cayenne Pepper

- Oregano Rosemary Celery Seed Thyme

- Tomato Paste Cilantro Basil

- Garlic Powder or Paste Mustard Powder

- Turmeric Red Pepper Onion Powder

- Worcestershire Sauce Horseradish Sauce

- Turmeric

## Proteins

- Boneless Chicken Breast
- Filet Mignon
- Sirloin
- Extra Lean Ground Beef
- Veal
- Organic Grass Fed Beef
- Buffalo
- Tilapia
- Grouper
- Cod
- Halibut
- Flounder
- Sole
- Sea Bass
- Shellfish
- Shrimp
- Lobster
- Crab
- Scallops

*Tip* Purchase all proteins raw and in bulk. Weigh and cut into (oz). (See Food Chart) individual portions. Cover with plastic wrap and place poultry, meat and fish in separate containers and store in freezer.

## Vegetables

- Asparagus

- Broccoli

- Cabbage

- Green Bell Pepper

- Brussels Sprouts

- Spinach

- Celery

- Cucumber

- Tomato

- White and Green Onions

- Green Leaf Lettuce

*Note- Fresh or frozen vegetables only, canned is prohibited (may contain added salt and preservatives).*

# Fruits

- ➲ Strawberries

- ➲ Oranges

- ➲ Grapefruit

- ➲ Green Apples

- ➲ Lemons

    *Note- Fresh or frozen fruit only, canned is prohibited (may contain added sugar and preservatives).*

## Beverages

- Bottled or Filtered Water

- Sparkling Mineral Water

- Herbal Teas (any tea bag assortment)

- Unsweetened Green Tea

- Unsweetened Black Tea

- Unsweetened Wu-Long Tea

- Coffee

- Non Dairy Unsweetened Soy Milk

- Fat Free Sugar Free Lucerne Coffee Creamer

# BEVERAGES RECIPES

## Frozen Mocha Cappuccino

- ➲ 1 C Crushed Ice

- ➲ 5 Drops of Chocolate Stevia

- ➲ 5 Drops of Valencia Orange

- ➲ 1 C of Black Coffee

- ➲ 1 Tbsp Lucerne Sugar Free Fat Free Coffee Creamer (2 tbsp allowed in 24 hr period)

    <u>Directions:</u> Mix in blender until smooth. Pour into glass and serve!

# Sparkling Lemonade

- 1 ½ Lemons (Juice)

- 2 Packages Stevia

- Sparkling Mineral Water

<u>Directions:</u> Pour lemon juice into 8 oz. glass. Add stevia, over ice and serve!

## Strawberry Slurpee

- 1 ½ Lemons (Juice)

- 1 Hand Full Strawberries

- 2 Packages Stevia

- 1 Sparkling Mineral Water

Directions: Pour lemon juice, strawberries and ice in blender pour into 8 oz. glass and serve with straw!

# Orange Julius

- 1 Orange

- 5-10 Drops Vanilla Crème Liquid Stevia

- Crushed Ice

- Bottled or Filtered Water (as needed)

  Directions: Peel orange and place orange sections in blender. Mix and serve.

# V-8 Tomato Juice

- 3 large Tomatoes

- Juice of Half a Lemon

- 1 tsp Cilantro

- ½ tsp Stevia

- ½ tsp Garlic Paste

- ¼ tsp Cumin

- ¼ tsp Braggs Pure Amino Acids

- 1/8 tsp Celery Seed

- Pinch of Sea Salt/Black Pepper

    Directions: In blender, combine all ingredients and puree until desired consistency. Place in refrigerator until chilled or serve over ice.

# EGG RECIPES

## Omelet

- 1 Whole Egg
- 3 Egg Whites
- 1 tsp Coconut Oil
- 1 to 2 Garlic Cloves (crushed)
- 1/3 Onion
- Handful of Broccoli
- Salt (to taste)
- Black Pepper (to taste)
- Cayenne Pepper (to taste)
- Paprika (to taste)

Directions: Sauté onion and garlic in 1/2 t coconut oil. Add broccoli and 1/4 cup of water. Cover and let steam until broccoli is a dark green and slightly crunchy. Remove from pan and set aside. Put the heat on low to medium heat, add 1/2 t of coconut oil. Tilt pan until oil has reached sides and bottom. Let oil heat for a minute or two. Pour on the eggs, spreading them evenly with a spatula. Tilt egg mixture until the liquid is no longer running onto sides. Cover and let set until there is no liquid left in the eggs. Remove eggs onto a plate. Place vegetables on top. Cover vegetables with eggs, like a sandwich. *I add hot sauce on top :)*

# Spanish Omelet

- One Whole Egg
- 3 Egg Whites
- ¼ cup chopped onion
- 5 asparagus spears
- 1 clove garlic
- 2 tsp coconut oil
- Salt and pepper
- Cayenne pepper to taste
- Salsa

# Egg Florentine

- 1 Whole Egg

- 3 Egg Whites

- 1 tsp Coconut Oil

- 1 to 2 Garlic Cloves (crushed)

- 1/3 Onion

- 2 Handfuls of Spinach

- Salt (to taste)

- Black Pepper (to taste)

- Cayenne Pepper (to taste)

- Paprika (to taste)

Directions: Sauté onion and garlic in 1t coconut oil. Add spinach. Stir until spinach cooks down. Add egg and seasonings. Scramble all ingredients until eggs are done. Enjoy.

## Chicken Broth

- 4.85 oz. Chicken Breast
- Parsley
- Onion Powder
- Garlic
- Thyme
- Rosemary
- Oregano
- Basil
- Bay Leaf
- Sea Salt
- Black Pepper

Directions: Fill saucepan 3/4 full with water. Bring to a boil. Add chicken and seasonings. Boil for 20 minutes. Remove boiled chicken and save for later. Strain out bay leaf & seasonings. Serve!

# Green Onion Soup

- ➲ Green Onions as Desired
- ➲ 2 C Bottled Water
- ➲ 2 tsp Liquid Aminos
- ➲ 1 tsp Parsley
- ➲ ½ tsp Paprika
- ➲ ½ tsp Sea Salt
- ➲ ½ tsp Dill
- ➲ ½ tsp Thyme
- ➲ 1/8 tsp Cayenne Pepper
- ➲ 1/8 tsp Celery Seed

Directions: Briefly steam the green onions until tender. Preheat saucepan over MED heat. Chop steamed green onions. Sauté green onions in saucepan with parsley, paprika, sea salt, dill, thyme, celery seed, liquid aminos and cayenne pepper. Add water and simmer 20-30 minutes and serve

## Turkey Meatball Soup

- 3.66 oz 93% Lean Ground Turkey or 5 oz. of 99% Lean Ground Turkey
- 1 tsp Coconut Oil
- 1 tsp Onion Powder
- 1 tsp Garlic Power
- 1 tbsp Cumin
- 1 tsp Cayenne Pepper (Optional)
- 1 tsp Paprika
- 1 Clove of Garlic
- 1 C Vegetable or Chicken Broth (zero calories)
- 1/2 C Water
- 1/3 White Onion
- 1 Italian Tomato
- 1 Tbsp Tomato Paste
- Salt and Pepper to taste
- Braggs to taste

Directions: Mix all seasonings with ground turkey. Form into little balls. Heat coconut oil in frying pan. Brown turkey balls (just on the outside, the middle should remain a little pink.) Remove turkey balls from frying pan and place in a sauce pan. Add broth, water, onion, tomato, tomato paste, Braggs and all the seasonings again. Bring to a boil. Cover and simmer for 30 minutes or longer. Turn heat off and let stand. Enjoy!  *You can use hamburger. Remember to reduce the ounces of hamburger.*

## Cucumber Salad

- 1 Cucumber

- 1 Tomato

- 1 Onion

- 1/2 C Apple Cider Vinegar

- Salt and Black Pepper to taste

Directions: Slice and quarter all ingredients. Combine and add salt, pepper and or cayenne pepper. The longer this salad marinates the better. I re-use the liquid as the vegetables are eaten and if necessary add more apple cider vinegar to taste.

## Green Salad

- ➲ 3 or 4 Leaves of Romaine

- ➲ Handful of Mixed lettuce

- ➲ 1/3 Onion

- ➲ 1 Tomato

- ➲ 1/2 Cucumber

Directions: Cut and combine.

# Cucumber-Tomato-and-Onion Salad

- 200 grams Thinly Sliced Cucumber (or allowed amount)

- 1 Medium Tomato

- ½ Chopped Onion

- 1 tsp Apple Cider Vinegar (to taste)

- 1 tsp Dill

- 2 tsp Melted Coconut Oil

- Brags Liquid Aminos (as needed)

- Black Pepper

- Sea Salt

Directions: Combine all ingredients -cucumber, tomatoes, and Onion & mix well. Toss in cucumbers. Cover & refrigerate. This tastes best if you wait at least one hour before serving.

# Apple Chicken Salad

- 4.85 oz. Diced Chicken Breast

- 4 diced Celery Stalks

- 4 Tbsp Lemon Juice

- Pinch of Cinnamon

- 1 package Stevia

- Squeeze of Lemon

- 1 Diced Green Apple

Directions: Mix ingredients together and serve!

# Taco Salad

- 3.66 oz 93% Lean Ground Turkey or 5 oz. of 99% Lean Ground Turkey
- 1 tsp Onion Powder
- 1 tsp Garlic Powder
- 1 Tbsp Cumin
- 1/2 tsp Oregano
- 1 Tbsp Cilantro
- 1 tsp Cayenne Pepper
- 1 tsp Paprika
- 1/2 Tbsp Chipotle Chili Pepper
- 1 tsp Jalapeno Pepper
- Braggs to taste

Directions: Brown Turkey and spices. Spray Braggs for moisture and to taste. You may add more of any spices you like for your taste. Half way through browning process adds ingredients below in order.

# Taco Salad (Cont'd)

- ➲ 1 C Vegetable or Chicken Broth (zero calories)
- ➲ 1/3 White Onion
- ➲ 1 Glove Garlic
- ➲ 1 Tbsp Cumin
- ➲ 1/2 tsp Oregano
- ➲ 1 Tbsp Cilantro
- ➲ 1 tsp Cayenne Pepper
- ➲ 1 tsp Paprika
- ➲ 1/2 Tbsp Chipotle Chili Pepper
- ➲ 1 tsp Jalapeno Pepper
- ➲ Braggs to taste ( I use Braggs in place of Salt)

  Bring to boil. Simmer for 15 minutes. I like my taco meat very spicy so I add a lot more of the spices above. Season to your personal taste.

- ➲ 1 Handful of Lettuce
- ➲ 1 Handful of Tomato
- ➲ 1 Handful of Onion (optional)
- ➲ Dressing - Cholula Hot Sauce or Tapatío (There are no calories in either so use as much as you want)

  Directions: Cut all ingredients and place on a plate. Make a bowl in the middle and place taco meat on top of salad. Enjoy!

## Shredded Chicken Taco Salad

- 4.85 oz Chicken Breast (Boiled, then shredded)
- 1 tsp Onion Powder
- 1 tsp Garlic Powder
- 1 C Vegetable or Chicken Broth (zero calories)
- 1/3 White Onion
- 1 Glove Garlic
- 1 Tbsp Cumin
- 1/2 tsp Oregano
- 1 Tbsp Cilantro
- 1 tsp Cayenne Pepper
- 1 tsp Paprika
- 1/2 Tbsp Chipotle Chili Pepper
- 1 tsp Jalapeno Pepper
- Braggs to taste ( I use Braggs in place of Salt)

Directions: Bring to boil. Simmer for 15 minutes. I like my taco meat very spicy so I add a lot more of the spices above. Season to your taste.

- 1 Handful of Lettuce
- 1 Handful of Tomato
- 1 Handful of Onion (optional)
- Dressing - Cholula Hot Sauce or Tapatío (There are no calories in either so use as much as you want)

Directions: Cut all ingredients and place on a plate. Make a bowl in the middle and place taco meat on top of salad. Enjoy!

# Vegetable Medley Saute

➲  1 to 3 Cloves of Garlic

➲  1/3 of Onion (Sliced)

➲  1 tsp Coconut Oil

➲  Handful of Broccoli

Sauté coconut oil, garlic and onion. When onion is clear add 1/8 or 1/4 water (any organic broth may be used as long as it has NO calories). Cover and let steam until broccoli is dark green. I like my vegetables crunchy. Steam longer if you want your vegetables soft. *YOU MAY USE ANY VEGTABLE OTHER THAN BROCCOLI AS LONG AS IT'S ON THE LIST OF FOODS ON PHASE II.*

# CHICKEN RECIPES

## Chicken "N" Broccoli

- ➲ 4.85 oz Chicken Breast
- ➲ 1 cup Broccoli
- ➲ 2 Tbsp Braggs Liquid Amino
- ➲ Sea Salt & Black Pepper
- ➲ 2 Cloves of Garlic
- ➲ ½ Chopped Onion
- ➲ Cayenne Pepper
- ➲ Chili Powder
- ➲ 2 tsp Organic Coconut Oil
- ➲ Juice from ½ Lemon

# Crock-Pot Chicken

- 6 Boneless Skinless Chicken Breasts

- 4 Onions cut into 1 inch pieces

- 1 Celery bunch, cut into 1 inch pieces

- 1 Head of garlic separated and peeled

- 2-3 cups of Water • Allowable Spices

Directions: In crock-pot, layer 1/2 celery, 1/2 onion, garlic pieces and chicken breasts. Sprinkle chicken with a layer of spices. Top with remaining celery and onion and another layer of spices. Add water almost to top. Cook on low for 8-9 hours. Weigh chicken and enjoy!

# Thai Chicken Wrap

- 1 Extra Large Iceberg Lettuce Leaf
- 4.85 oz. Boneless Skinless Chicken Breast
- 1/4 cup White Onions, Diced
- 1/4 cup Green Peppers, Diced
- 3 Cherry Tomatoes, Diced
- Pinch of Black Pepper
- Pinch of Sea Salt

Directions: Chop chicken breast into small square pieces. Cook chicken, onions and green peppers in pan. Place on top of lettuce leaf. Add diced tomatoes and season with black pepper and sea salt. Fold leaf lettuce in half and serve!

# Ginger Chicken

- ➲ 3 1/2 oz. Chicken Breast

- ➲ 3 Stalks Celery

- ➲ 3 Tbsp Blue Agave

- ➲ 2 Tbsp Liquid Amino Marinade

- ➲ 2 tsp Ground Ginger

Directions: Chop celery and sauté in pan. Cook half way through then add chicken, adding just enough water through-out cooking to maintain food so it will not burn. When finished, add all ingredients and let it caramelize slowly over low heat.

# Curry Chicken

- 4.85 oz. Chicken Breasts
- 1 C Vegetable or Chicken Broth (Organic no calories)
- 1 tsp Coconut Oil
- 1/3 White Onion
- 1 to 2 Cloves of Garlic
- 2 Tbsp Curry Powder
- 1/2 tsp Turmeric
- 1/4 tsp Black Pepper
- 1/2 tsp Paprika
- 1 tsp Cumin
- 1/2 tsp Ginger
- 1/2 tsp Cayenne pepper (optional)
- Braggs to taste

Directions: Cut chicken breasts into small squares. Put coconut oil in a frying pan and brown outside of chicken only (should be real pink inside) Add vegetable broth, water, onion, garlic and spices. Bring to boil. Simmer on low for 20 to 30 minutes. Then cover and let set for another 20 to 30 minutes. You may add more spices if desired.

# SEAFOOD RECIPES

## Shrimp Cocktail

- ➲ 5 oz. Shrimp (Peeled and Deveined)
- ➲ 6 oz. Tomato Paste
- ➲ 1 Tbsp Braggs Pure Amino Acids
- ➲ 1 Tbsp Lemon Juice
- ➲ ½ tsp Celery Seed
- ➲ 2 Tbsp Chopped Parsley
- ➲ Pinch of Cayenne Pepper
- ➲ Pinch of Black Pepper
- ➲ Pinch of Sea Salt
- ➲ Pinch of Cumin

Directions: Mix ingredients together, add shrimp, chill and serve!

# Scallops

- 6 oz. Scallops

- 1 to 2 Cloves of Garlic (Minced)

- 1 slice of Onion

- 1/2 tsp Cayenne pepper

- 1 tsp Cumin

- 1/4 tsp Black Pepper

- 1/2 tsp Turmeric

- 1/2 tsp Paprika

- Braggs to taste ( I use Braggs in place of Salt)

- 1 Handful of Broccoli or Green Beans

- 1 tsp Coconut Oil

Directions: Heat 1 tsp of coconut oil in pan. Sauté garlic and onion. When onion is clear add scallops and all seasonings. You may add or subtract any of the seasonings as you wish. Sear the scallops on all sides. There should be juices from the scallops, then add your broccoli or green beans and spray with Braggs. If you wish you may add more seasonings at this time. Mix all ingredients and cover for 3 to 5 minutes. *Serve with Cucumber Salad or Green Salad.*

# Shrimp Scampi

- 5 oz. Peeled Shrimp

- 2 Cloves Garlic (crushed)

- 1/3 Onion, sliced

- Salt to taste

- Black Pepper to taste

- 1/4 tsp Parsley

- 1/8 tsp Red Pepper Flakes

- Handful of Broccoli

- Lemon Juice from half a Lemon. Just one squeeze.

   Directions: In a heavy-bottomed pan, melt coconut oil over medium-low heat. Add the garlic and onion. Sauté for 1 minute; be careful, the garlic burns easily! Add the shrimp, salt, pepper, parsley, red pepper flakes and paprika. Sauté until the shrimp have just turned pink, about 3 to 4 minutes, stirring often. You may want to add a little water. Add broccoli and lemon juice. Cover and let steam for 3 to 4 minutes. Broccoli should be dark green and moderately what crispy. *Serve with Cucumber Salad or Green Salad.*

# Grilled Chilean Sea Bass

- 5.8 oz. Chilean Sea Bass

- 1 tsp Onion Powder

- 1 tsp Garlic Powder

- 1 tbsp Cumin

- 1 tsp Cayenne Pepper (Optional)

- 1 tsp Paprika

- 1/4 of Green Cabbage

- 1/4 to 1/2 C Salsa (Make sure the salsa has only the ingredients allowed. I use one from Whole Foods)

Directions: Season Chilean sea bass with onion, garlic powder, cumin, cayenne pepper and paprika. Grill on BBQ or George Forman Grill. You will know it's done when the fish is white in the middle. This fish is VERY hard to burn. Steam green cabbage. Place cabbage on plate and top with salsa. *Serve with Cucumber Salad or Green Salad.*

# Halibut Wrapped

- ⮑ 4.85 oz. of Halibut

- ⮑ 1 tsp Onion Powder

- ⮑ 1 tsp Garlic Powder

- ⮑ 1 Tbsp Cumin

- ⮑ 1 tsp Cayenne Pepper (Optional)

- ⮑ 1 tsp Paprika

- ⮑ 1 tsp Coconut Oil

- ⮑ 1 to 3 Cloves of Garlic

- ⮑ 1/3 of Onion (sliced)

- ⮑ Handful of any one or two vegetables

- ⮑ Aluminum Foil to wrap all Ingredients

Directions: Preheat oven to 400 degrees. Sprinkle seasonings on fish. Place seasoned fish, garlic, onion, and vegetables in foil. Melt coconut oil and dribble on top. Wrap tightly then place on cookie sheet or casserole pan. Bake for 30 to 40 minutes or until fish is flaky. You might want to check fish every 15 minutes. *Serve with cucumber salad or green salad.*

*\*YOU CAN USE ANY FISH ON THE LIST IN PLACE OF HALIBUT. OUNCES WILL VARY.*

# TURKEY & BEEF RECIPES

## Turkey Burger

- 3.66 oz 93% Lean Ground Turkey or 5 oz. of 99% Lean Ground Turkey
- 1 tsp Onion Powder
- 1 tsp Garlic Powder
- 1 Tbsp Cumin
- 1 tsp Cayenne Pepper (Optional)
- 1 tsp Paprika
- 1 Clove of Garlic
- Salt and Pepper to taste

  Directions: Roll turkey into balls then flatten slightly. Grill on BBQ or George Forman Grill.

- 2 to 3 Large Romaine Lettuce Leafs
- 1/2 Italian Tomato Sliced
- 1/4 Thick Onion Slice
- Mustard (Zero Calorie)
- Ketchup (see recipe)

  Directions: Cut the turkey burger in half then lay on one leaf of romaine. Add your tomato, onion, mustard and ketchup. Cover with other leaf, like a long hamburger bun :) *Serve with Cucumber Salad or Green Salad.*

# Turkey Chili

- 3.66 oz 93% Lean Ground Turkey or 5 oz. of 99% Lean Ground Turkey
- 1 tsp Onion Powder
- 1 tsp Garlic Powder
- 1 to 2 Tbsp Chili Pepper
- 1 Tbsp Cumin
- 1 Tbsp Cilantro
- 1 Tbsp Cayenne Pepper
- 1 tsp Paprika
- 1/2 Tbsp Chipotle Chili Pepper
- 1 tsp Jalapeno Pepper
- Braggs to taste

  Directions: Brown Turkey and spices. Spray Braggs for moisture and to taste. You may add more of any spices you like for your taste. Half way through browning process add ingredients listed below in order.

- 1 C Organic Vegetable or Chicken Broth (zero calories)
- 1 Italian Tomato Diced
- 1/3 White Onion
- 1 Glove Garlic
- 1 Tbsp Cumin
- 1 Tbsp Chili Pepper

- 1/2 tsp Oregano

- 1 Tbsp Cilantro

- 1 tsp Cayenne Pepper

- 1 tsp Paprika

- 1/2 Tbsp Chipotle Chili Pepper (Optional)

- 1 tsp Jalapeno Pepper (Optional)

- Braggs to taste ( I use Braggs in place of Salt)

   Directions: Bring to boil. Cover and simmer for 30 minutes to 1 hour. I like my chili very spicy so I add a lot more of the spices above. Season to your taste.

# Hamburger

- 3.95 oz of 95% Lean Hamburger

- 1 tsp Onion Powder

- 1 tsp Garlic Powder

- 1 Tbsp Cumin

- 1 tsp Cayenne Pepper (Optional)1 tsp Paprika

- Salt and Pepper to taste

    Direction: Roll hamburger into balls then flatten slightly. Grill on BBQ or George Forman Grill.

- 2 to 3 Large Romaine Lettuce Leafs

- 1/2 Italian Tomato Sliced

- 1/4 Thick Onion Slice

- Mustard (Zero Calorie)

- Ketchup (see recipe)

    Direction: I cut the hamburger burger in half then lay on one leaf of romaine. Add your tomato, onion mustard and ketchup. Cover with other leaf, like a long hamburger bun :) *Serve with Cucumber Salad or Green Salad*

# DESSERTS

## Lemonade

- 1 Lemon (Juice)
- 2 Vanilla Stevia's
- 8 oz. Sparkling Water

  Directions: Squeeze juice from one lemon. Add stevia, water and ice.

## Lemonade, Strawberry Slushy

- ➲ 1 Lemon (Juice)
- ➲ 2 Vanilla Stevia's
- ➲ 5 Strawberry's
- ➲ 8 oz. Sparkling Water
- ➲ Ice

Directions: Use blender to mix all ingredient.

# Hot Apple Pie

- 1 Apple
- 1 Vanilla Stevia
- Cinnamon to taste

Directions: Cut apple in bit size pieces. Add vanilla stevia and cinnamon. Microwave for 30 seconds; If you want your apples softer and hotter, microwave longer. I like my apples crunchy.

# Apple Pie

- 1 Apple

- 1 Vanilla Stevia

- Cinnamon to taste

    <u>Directions:</u> Cut apple in bite size pieces. Add vanilla stevia and cinnamon.

# Strawberry and Apple Sweetness

- ➲ Handful of Strawberry's

- ➲ 1 Apple

- ➲ 1 to 2 packets of Vanilla Stevia

    <u>Directions:</u> Cut apple and strawberries into bite size pieces. Sprinkle vanilla stevia on top and mix.
    * This will count as 2 fruits

# How to Feel Good Naked IN 26 Days!
## With

# HCG Body 4 LIFE
# Phase III Recipes

## In Phase III

*You'll Burn the Fat and Reveal the Muscle*

# A Message from the Authors

*"One of the fastest ways to get what you want is to help other people get what THEY want." Author unknown....*That is one of the MANY reasons Colin and I wrote this recipe book for

Phase III.

I have to say this was the most fun to write. I have enjoyed all the experiments with different foods, seasonings, and herbs with no sugar or starches. One might think it would be difficult, but I'm here to tell you it's NOT!!!!

Several of our recipes are desserts. My down fall has always been treats, sugary, rich treats....Well I didn't let phase III stop me :) As you will see, chocolate is one of the many key ingredients to our most popular dessert recipes.

Hope you like chocolate.

In phase 2 my creativity was restricted and limited when it came to creating new and different recipes. As you may have noticed, the food choices are very limited. However, in Phase III the most of the limitation are lifted therefore, I was able to be more creative and so will the recipes to follow.

"Your time is limited, so don't waste it living someone else's life. Don't be trapped by dogma - which is living with the results of other people's thinking. Don't let the noise of others' opinions drown out your own inner voice; and most important, have the courage to follow your heart and intuition. They somehow already know what you truly want to become. Everything else is secondary."

**Steve Jobs**

# BREAKFAST

## PHASE III

### Greek Yogurt with Banana and Peanut Butter

- ⮂ 1/2 C Greek Yogurt
- ⮂ 1/2 Banana
- ⮂ 1 tsp. Peanut Butter
- ⮂ 2 Packets of Vanilla Stevia

Directions: Mix all together and enjoy.

*Calories: 275*

# Greek Yogurt with Fruit

➲ 1/2 C Greek Yogurt

➲ 2 Packets of Vanilla Stevia

➲ Fruit of Choice

Directions: Mix all together and enjoy.

*Calories:* 180

# Chocolate Greek Yogurt with Banana and Peanut Butter

- ➲  1/2 C Greek Yogurt

- ➲  1/2 Banana

- ➲  1 tsp. Peanut Butter

- ➲  1 to 2 tbsp. Chocolate Pudding

- ➲  2 Packets of Vanilla Stevia

   Directions: Mix all together and enjoy. *See Recipe for Chocolate Pudding

   *Calories: 354*

# Lemon Greek Yogurt with Blueberry's

- 1/2 C Greek Yogurt

- 2 to 3 tbsp Lemon Pudding

- 2 Packets of Vanilla Stevia

  Directions: Mix All together and enjoy *See Recipe for Lemon Pudding.

  *Calories:* 104

# Egg Skillet

- 3 Eggs
- 5 Egg Whites
- 1 T Coconut Oil
- 3 to 4 Strips of Prepared Bacon
- 1/2 C Broccoli
- 1/2 Zucchini
- 1/3 of Onion
- 2 to 3 Cloves of Garlic
- 1/2 of Red, Yellow, Orange or Green Pepper
- 2 to 3 Mushrooms Sliced
- 1/4 C Water
- 1/2 C. Any Cheese
- Salt (to taste)
- Black Pepper (to taste)
- Cayenne Pepper (to taste)
- Paprika (to taste)

Directions: Heat oven to 425 degrees.

Prepare bacon and set aside. Sauté onion and garlic and coconut oil in a wrought iron skillet. Add all vegetables and water, stir, cover and let steam for 2 to 3 minutes. Add eggs (whisked) and scramble all ingredients for 2 to 3 minutes. The egg mixture should be a little wet. Place entire skillet into the oven with cheese sprinkled on top. Bake for 10 to 15 minutes. Eggs should be white and cheese melted.

* You can use any vegetables, seasonings or herbs.

*Calories: 266 per serving (4 servings)*

# Omelet

- 1 Whole Egg

- 4 Egg Whites

- 1 to 2 tsp. Coconut Oil

- 1 to 2 Garlic Cloves (crushed)

- 1/3 Onion

- 1/2 C Broccoli

- 1/2 C Red, Yellow, Orange or Green Bell Pepper

- 2 Mushrooms sliced

- 1 to 2 oz. Any Cheese

- Salt (to taste)

- Black Pepper (to taste)

- Cayenne Pepper (to taste)

- Paprika (to taste)

Directions: Sauté onion and garlic in 1 tsp. coconut oil. Add broccoli, bell pepper, mushrooms and 1/4 cup of water. Cover and let steam until broccoli is a dark green and slightly crunchy. Remove from pan and set aside.

Put the heat on low to medium heat; add 1 tsp. of coconut oil. Tilt pan until oil has reached sides and bottom. Let oil heat for a minute or two. Pour on the eggs, spreading them evenly with a spatula. Tilt egg mixture until the liquid is no longer running onto sides. Cover and let set until there is no liquid left in the eggs. Remove eggs onto a plate. Place vegetables on top along with cheese. Cover vegetables with eggs, like a sandwich.

*I add hot sauce or salsa on top :)

_Calories:_ 444

## Spanish Omelet

- 1 Whole Egg
- 4 Egg Whites
- 1 to 2 tsp. Coconut Oil
- 1 to 2 Garlic Cloves (crushed)
- 1/3 Onion
- 1/2 C Red, Yellow, Orange or Green Bell Pepper
- 2 Mushrooms sliced
- 1/2 Jalapeno Pepper sliced and remove seeds (optional)
- Green Chilies to taste
- 1 C Turkey Chili (see recipe)
- 1 to 2 oz. Any Cheese
- Salt (to taste)
- Black Pepper (to taste)
- Cayenne Pepper (to taste)
- Paprika (to taste)

Directions: Sauté onion and garlic in 1t coconut oil. Add bell pepper, mushrooms, jalapeno pepper, chilies and 1/4 cup of water. Cover and let steam until vegetables are slightly crunchy. Remove from pan and set aside.

Put the heat on low to medium heat, add 1t of coconut oil. Tilt pan until oil has reached sides and bottom. Let oil heat for a minute or two. Pour on the eggs, spreading them evenly with a spatula. Tilt egg mixture until the liquid is no longer running onto sides. Cover and let set until there is no liquid left in the eggs. Remove eggs onto a plate. Place vegetables on top along with turkey chili and cheese. Cover vegetables with eggs, like a sandwich.

*I add hot sauce or salsa on top :)

*Calories: 528*

# Egg Florentine

- 1 Whole Egg
- 4 Egg Whites
- 1 to 2 tsp. Coconut Oil
- 1 to 2 Garlic Cloves (crushed)
- 1/3 Onion
- 2 Handfuls of Spinach
- 2 Mushrooms sliced
- 1 to 2 oz. White Cheese
- Salt (to taste)
- Black Pepper (to taste)
- Cayenne Pepper (to taste)
- Paprika (to taste)

Directions: Sauté onion and garlic in 1t coconut oil. Add spinach and mushrooms. Stir until spinach cooks down. Add egg and seasonings. Scramble all ingredients until eggs are done. Top with cheese and enjoy.

*Calories:* 356 (1 oz. cheese)

# MAIN COURSE

## PHASE III

### Turkey Chili

- ➲ 1 lb Lean Turkey

- ➲ 1 tbsp Onion Powder

- ➲ 2 tsp. Garlic Powder

- ➲ 1 tbsp Chili Powder

- ➲ Braggs to taste

  <u>Directions:</u> Brown Turkey and spices. Spray Braggs for moisture and to taste. You may add more of any spices you like for your taste. Add ingredients below half way through browning process (In the order listed).

- ➲ 1 15 oz. Tomato Sauce (organic no sugar added)

- ➲ 1 to 2 tbsp Tomato Paste (organic no sugar added)

- ➲ 2 - 3 Chipotle Peppers in Adobo Sauce

- ➲ 1 tbsp Adobo Sauce

- ➲ 1 C Vegetable Broth

- ➲ 1 C Water

- ➲ 1/2 to 1 Whole White Onion

- ➲ 1/2 Red Pepper

- 1/2 Yellow Pepper

- 5 Cloves Garlic

- 2 to 4 Tomatoes

- 1 tbsp Chili Powder

- 1 tsp. Cayenne pepper

- 2 tsp. Cumin

- 1/4 tsp. Black Pepper

- 1 tsp. Turmeric

- 1 tsp. Paprika

- Braggs to taste ( I use Braggs in place of Salt)

  Directions: Bring to boil. Cover and simmer for 30 minutes to 1 hour. I like my chili very spicy so I add a lot more of the spices above. Season according to your own taste.

  *Calories: 107 per serving (10 servings)*

# Chicken BBQ in Slow Cooker

- 13 oz. BBQ Sauce (Organic Ville from Whole Foods or BBQ sauce without sugar)
- 1/2 C Italian Dressing (365 Organic from Whole Foods or no sugar)
- Braggs to taste
- Liquid Smoke to taste
- 3 Chipotle Chilies
- 1 tbsp Adobo Sauce from Chipotle Chili's
- 6 Chicken Breast no skin

Directions:U Combine all ingredients in slow cooker and allow cooking on high for 8 or more hours.

*Calories: 392*

# Curry Chicken

- 2 Skinless Chicken Breasts
- 1 C Vegetable Broth (Organic)
- 1 C Coconut Milk (Organic)
- 1 tsp. Coconut Oil
- 1 White Onion
- 5 Cloves of Garlic
- 2 tbsp Curry Powder
- 1 tsp. Turmeric
- 1 tsp. Paprika
- 1 tsp. Cumin
- 1/2 tsp. Ginger
- 1/2 tsp. Cayenne Pepper (optional)
- Braggs to taste

Directions: Cut chicken breasts into small squares. Put coconut oil in a frying pan and brown outside of chicken only (should be real pink inside) Add vegetable broth, coconut milk, onion, garlic and spices. Bring to boil. Simmer on low for 20 to 30 minutes. Then cover and let set for another 20 to 30 minutes. You may add more spices if desired.

*Calories: 129 per serving (10 servings)*

## Salmon Wraps

- 6 oz. Canned Salmon

- 1 to 2 T Organic Mayonnaise

- 1/4 C Salsa or Hot Sauce to taste

- 1 1/4 inch slice Onion

- Salt to taste or Braggs

- Black Pepper to taste

- Cayenne Pepper (optional)

- 4 small Romaine Lettuce Leaves

- 1 oz. Monterey Jack Cheese

Directions: Combine salmon, Braggs, mayonnaise, salt, pepper, cayenne pepper, salsa or hot sauce or both :) and onion. Place a little in each lettuce leaf. Garnish with tomato and Monterey jack cheese...Eat up :)

*Calories: 405*

## Zero Pasta Lasagna

*If you didn't want to go through the task of making your own sauce, this recipe could easily be put together with a healthy no-sugar-added jar of marinara sauce.

- 1 pound Spicy Chicken Sausage
- 1 pound Ground Turkey
- ½ Cup Minced Onion
- 5 Cloves Garlic, Crushed
- 1 (32 oz.) Can Tomato Sauce
- 1/2 (6 oz.) Can Tomato Paste
- 3 Cups Chicken Broth
- 1/2 Onion
- 1 Red Bell Pepper
- 1 ½ tsp. dried basil leaves
- 1 tsp. Italian Seasoning
- 1 TBS Celtic Sea Salt
- ¼ tsp. Ground Black Pepper
- 4 TBS Chopped Fresh Parsley
- 1/2 Head of Cabbage
- 16 oz. Ricotta Cheese
- 1 Egg

- ½ tsp. Salt

- ¾ lb. Mozzarella Cheese Grated

- ¾ Cup Parmesan Cheese

Directions: Boil water in a large pot. Clean cabbage and gently peel leaves. Place in water, boil for 5 minutes or until soft and tender...they won't soften when you cook the lasagna. Remove from water and drain.

Preheat oven to 425 degrees. In a Dutch oven, cook sausage, ground beef, onion, and garlic over medium heat until well browned. Stir in crushed tomatoes, tomato sauce. Season with stevia, basil, fennel seeds, Italian seasoning, 1 tablespoon salt, pepper, and 2 TBS parsley. Simmer covered, for about 1 1/2 hours, stirring occasionally. In a mixing bowl, combine ricotta cheese with egg, remaining parsley, and 1/2 tsp. salt. Preheat oven to 375 degrees.

To assemble, spread 1 1/2 cups of meat sauce in the bottom of a 9x13 inch baking dish. Arrange cabbage noodles lengthwise over meat sauce. Spread with one half of the ricotta cheese mixture. Top with a third of mozzarella cheese slices.

Spoon 1 1/2 cups meat sauce over mozzarella, and sprinkle with 1/4 cup Parmesan cheese. Repeat layers, and top with remaining mozzarella and Parmesan cheese. Cover with foil: to prevent sticking, either spray foil with cooking spray, or make sure the foil does not touch the cheese. Bake for 25 minutes. Remove foil, and bake an additional 25 minutes. Cool for 15 minutes before serving.

*Calories: 275 per serving (12servings)*

# Enchiladas

- 1 Pound Chicken Sausage
- 1 Pound Ground Turkey
- 1 to 2 TBS Cumin (to taste)
- 1 to 2 TBS Chili Pepper (to taste)
- Salt to taste
- 1 tsp. Cheyenne Pepper
- 1 C Cheddar Cheese (Grated)
- 1 C Pepper Jack (Optional)
- 1/2 Onion (Diced)
- 1 (32 oz.) Can Enchilada Sauce
- Tooth Picks

Directions: Boil water in a large pot. Clean cabbage and gently peel leaves. Place in water, boil for 5 minutes or until soft and tender...they won't soften when you cook the lasagna. Remove from water and drain.

Preheat oven to 375 degrees.
Cook sausage, ground turkey and all seasonings, over medium heat until well browned. Place grated cheeses, onion and enchilada sauce in separate containers creating an assembly line. Dip cabbage leaf into enchilada sauce, then stuff chicken sausage, turkey, cheese and onion into cabbage leaf. Roll and secure with tooth pick. Stuff each cabbage leaf until your ingredients are gone. Pour remaining enchilada sauce on top of enchilada's and top with cheese. Spray aluminum foil with Pam. Cover enchiladas and bake for 30 minutes. Remove foil, bake until cheese is brown and sauce is bubbling.

*Calories: 181 per serving (16 Serving)*

# Stuffed Greek Chicken

- 4 skinless, boneless chicken breasts
- Small Package of Feta Cheese
- Package of Fresh Basil
- 8 to 10 Sun Dried Tomatoes
- 3 Cloves Garlic
- 1/4 C. Chopped Onion
- 2 to 3 C. Chicken Broth
- 2 TBS Italian Seasoning
- 1/4 C. Braggs Amino Acid
- 1 to 2 TBS Olive Oil

Directions: Sprinkle chicken with Italian seasoning. Using a small sharp knife, cut in half horizontally through the center of each chicken breast half, creating a pocket. Fill each pocket with 2 sun dried tomatoes, 2 to 3 fresh basil leaves and 1 TBS of feta cheese. Roll and close with a tooth pick.

In a large skillet sauté garlic and onion in olive oil over medium heat. Add filled, chicken breast halves to skillet and sauté until outsides are golden brown. Insides should be pink. Add chicken broth and Braggs. Simmer chicken until fully cooked. Juices should run clear. Approximately 5 minutes.

*Calories: 287 per serving (4 servings)*

## BREAD & CHIPS

# PHASE III

### Low Carb Flax Bread

- ⮑ 1/3 C Flax Seed Oil or Coconut Oil
- ⮑ 1/2 C Water
- ⮑ 1 tsp. Salt
- ⮑ 1 Packet Stevia
- ⮑ 1 tbsp Baking Powder
- ⮑ 2 Eggs
- ⮑ 4 Egg Whites
- ⮑ 2 C Flax Seed Meal (You can find this at most grocery stores or grind whole flax seeds into a meal)

Directions: Preheat the oven to 350 degrees. In large bowl, mix flax seed meal, stevia, salt and baking powder. Whisk oil, water and eggs (In a separate bowl). Combine all ingredients and let set for 2 to 3 minutes until thick.

Place oiled parchment paper on baking sheet. Pour batter onto the baking sheet. Once you have it all there, you can spread this out on your baking sheet to whatever thickness you desire, but it should be at least 1/2 inch thick.

Place into preheated oven for about 25 minutes. You want to push on the bread and if it bounces back a bit it is done. Let cool for about 25 minutes.

NOTE: This is the basic bread recipe. You can add any ingredient you like. I add sun dried tomatoes and basil. Also, I add 1 banana and substitute 1 cup of apple sauce for oil. PLAY! :)

Calories: 118 per serving (12 Servings)

## Flax Seed Chips

- 1/2 C Flax Seeds

- 1/2 C Flax Meal

- 6 Medium Tomatoes

- 1 C Sun-Dried Tomatoes

- 1 tbsp Lemon Juice

- 1/4 C Fresh Basil

- 3 Medium Onions

- 1 Clove Garlic

- 1 tbsp Braggs

Directions: Grind all ingredients in a food processor. Spread evenly and thinly over 2 Para flex dehydrator trays, right to the edges. Dehydrate at 105 degrees for 3 hours then invert onto another mesh dehydrator tray to finish drying in the dehydrator for a further 10 – 18 hours.

* If you like it spicy, add a habanera and cayenne pepper to taste.

Calories: 42 per chip (20 chips)

## SAUCES

# PHASE III

### Pesto

- 2/3 C Walnuts or Pine Nuts

- 6 Sun Dried Tomatoes

- 20 Basil Leaves

- 1 tbsp Olive Oil or Flax Seed Oil

- 2 Garlic Cloves

- Braggs to taste

Directions: Combine all ingredients into food processor. Add any one or all ingredients to taste. I like to add a habanera pepper.

Calories: 61 per tablespoon (16 tablespoons)

## Cilantro Pesto

- 2/3 C Walnuts or Pine Nuts

- 1 Bunch of Cilantro

- 1 tbsp Olive Oil or Flax Seed Oil

- 3 Garlic Cloves

- 1 Tomato

- 5 Sun dried Tomatoes

- Braggs to Taste

- 1 Hot Pepper (Optional)

Directions: Combine all ingredients into food processor. Add a little water if too thick. Add one or all of the above ingredients to taste.

*Calories: 61 per tablespoon (16 tablespoons)*

# DRESSING AND SAUCES

**Braggs**

**Lemon Juice of one Lemon**

**Apple Cider Vinegar**

**Braggs and 1 tsp. Coconut Oil**

**Braggs and 1 tablespoons MTC Oil add tablespoon of Dijon Mustard**

## Ketchup

- 1/4 C Tomato Sauce (Organic no sugar added)
- 1/8 C Tomato Paste (Organic no sugar added)
- 1/2 tsp. Distilled White Vinegar
- 1/4 tsp. Sea Salt
- 1/2 tsp. Paprika
- 1/2 tsp. Onion Powder
- 1/2 tsp. Stevia

Directions: Combine all ingredients and enjoy. Mix well. * You may add or take away from seasoning to your liking. Also, I add garlic powder and Cheyenne pepper...but you know me :)

Calories: 61 per tablespoon (16 tablespoons)

# SALADS

## Mozzarella Italian Salad

- ⮑ 2 sticks String Cheese

- ⮑ 1/2 Cucumber Cubed

- ⮑ 1/2 Red Bell Pepper

- ⮑ 1 Large Tomato Sliced

- ⮑ 3 large Slices of Onion

- ⮑ 2 tablespoons Boursin Garlic Herb Cheese

- ⮑ 8 tablespoons Balsamic Vinegar

- ⮑ 1 tablespoon Olive Oil

Directions: Mix all ingredients together and let marinate for an hour or two.

*Calories: 112 (4 servings)*

## Mustard Brussels Sprout

- 16 Brussels sprouts

- 2 cloves garlic, crushed

- ½ tablespoons Cayenne Pepper

- 2 tablespoons Dijon Mustard

- 1 tablespoon Lemon Juice

- Salt and Ground Black pepper to taste

Directions: Place a steamer insert into a saucepan, and fill with water to just below the bottom of the steamer. Cover, and bring the water to a boil over high heat. Add the Brussels sprouts, and season with garlic and cayenne pepper. Recover, and steam to your desired degree of tenderness, about 30 minutes for very tender.

Remove the Brussels sprouts from the steamer and place into a bowl. Add the mustard, and lemon juice. Season to taste with salt and pepper toss until evenly coated.

*Calories:* *128 per serving (2 serving)*

## Cucumber Salad

- ⮑ 1 Cucumber

- ⮑ 1 Tomato

- ⮑ 1 Onion

- ⮑ 1/2 C Apple Cider Vinegar

- ⮑ Salt and Black Pepper to taste

Directions: Slice and quarter all ingredients. Combine and add salt, pepper and or cayenne pepper. The longer this salad marinates the better. I re-use the liquid as the vegetables are eaten and if necessary add more apple cider vinegar to taste.

# Green Salad

- 3 or 4 Leaves of Romaine
- Handful of Mixed lettuce
- 1/3 Onion
- 1 Tomato
- 1/2 Cucumber

Directions: Cut and combine.

# Taco Salad

- 3.66 oz 93% Lean Ground Turkey or 5 oz. of 99% Lean Ground Turkey
- 1 tsp. Onion Powder
- 1 tsp. Garlic Powder
- 1 tbsp Cumin
- 1/2 tsp. Oregano
- 1 tbsp Cilantro
- 1 tsp. Cayenne Pepper
- 1 tsp. Paprika
- 1/2 tbsp Chipotle Chili Pepper
- 1 tsp. Jalapeno Pepper
- Braggs to taste

  Directions: Brown Turkey and spices. Spray Braggs for moisture and to taste. You may add more of any spices you like for your taste. Add ingredients below in order listed half way through browning process.

- 1 C Vegetable or Chicken Broth (zero calories)
- 1/3 White Onion
- 1 Glove Garlic
- 1 tbsp Cumin
- 1/2 tsp. Oregano
- 1 tbsp Cilantro

- ⊃ 1 tsp. Cayenne Pepper

- ⊃ 1 tsp. Paprika

- ⊃ 1/2 tbsp Chipotle Chili Pepper

- ⊃ 1 tsp. Jalapeno Pepper

- ⊃ Braggs to taste ( I use Braggs in place of Salt)

  <u>Directions:</u> Bring to boil. Simmer for 15 minutes. I like my taco meat very spicy so I add a lot more of the spices above. Season to your personal taste.

- ⊃ 1 Handful of Lettuce

- ⊃ 1 Handful of Tomato1 Handful of Onion (optional)
- ⊃ Dressing - Cholula Hot Sauce or Tapatío (There are no calories in either so use as much as you want)

  <u>Directions:</u> Cut all ingredients and place on a plate. Make a bowl in the middle and place taco meat on top of salad. Enjoy!

## Shredded Chicken Taco Salad

- ➲ 4.85 Chicken Breast (boiled, then shredded)
- ➲ 1 tsp. Onion Powder
- ➲ 1 tsp. Garlic Powder
- ➲ 1 C Vegetable or Chicken Broth (zero calories)
- ➲ 1/3 White Onion
- ➲ 1 Glove Garlic
- ➲ 1 tbsp Cumin
- ➲ 1/2 tsp. Oregano
- ➲ 1 tbsp Cilantro
- ➲ 1 tsp. Cayenne Pepper
- ➲ 1 tsp. Paprika
- ➲ 1/2 tbsp Chipotle Chili Pepper
- ➲ 1 tsp. Jalapeno Pepper
- ➲ Braggs to taste ( I use Braggs in place of Salt)

Directions: Bring to boil. Simmer for 15 minutes. I like my taco meat very spicy so I add a lot more of the spices above. Season to your personal taste.

- ➲ 1 Handful of Lettuce
- ➲ 1 Handful of Tomato
- ➲ 1 Handful of Onion (optional)

Dressing - Cholula Hot Sauce or Tapatío (There are no calories in either so use as much as you want)
Directions: Cut all ingredients and place on a plate. Make a bowl in the middle and place taco meat on top of salad. Enjoy!

## Shrimp Scampi

- ➲ 5 oz. Peeled Shrimp

- ➲ 2 Cloves Garlic (crushed)

- ➲ 1/3 Onion, sliced

- ➲ Salt to taste

- ➲ Black Pepper to taste

- ➲ 1/4 tsp. Parsley

- ➲ 1/8 tsp. Red Pepper Flakes

- ➲ Handful of Broccoli

- ➲ Lemon Juice from half a Lemon. Just one squeeze

Directions:U In a heavy-bottomed pan, melt coconut oil over medium-low heat. Add the garlic and onion. Sauté for 1 minute; be careful, the garlic burns easily! Add the shrimp, salt, pepper, parsley, red pepper flakes and paprika. Sauté until the shrimp have just turned pink, about 3 to 4 minutes, stirring often. You may want to add a little water. Add broccoli and lemon juice. Cover and let steam for 3 to 4 minutes. Broccoli should be dark green and moderately crispy. Serve with Salad

# Grilled Chilean Sea Bass

- ⮫ 5.8 oz Chilean Sea Bass

- ⮫ 1 tsp. Onion Powder

- ⮫ 1 tsp. Garlic Powder

- ⮫ 1 tbsp Cumin

- ⮫ 1 tsp. Cayenne Pepper (Optional)

- ⮫ 1 tsp. Paprika

- ⮫ 1/4 of Green Cabbage

- ⮫ ¼ to ½ C Salsa (Make sure the salsa has only the ingredients allowed. I use one from Whole Foods)

Directions: Season Chilean sea bass with onion, garlic powder, cumin, cayenne pepper and paprika. Grill on BBQ or George Forman. You will know it's done when the fish is white in the middle. This fish is VERY hard to burn. Steam green cabbage. Place cabbage on plate and top with salsa.

# Turkey Burger

- 3.66 oz. 93% Lean Ground Turkey or 5 oz. of 99% Lean Ground Turkey

- 1 tsp. Onion Powder

- 1 tsp. Garlic Powder

- 1 tbsp Cumin

- 1 tsp. Cayenne Pepper (Optional)

- 1 tsp. Paprika

- 1 Clove of Garlic

- Salt and Pepper to taste

  Directions: Roll turkey into balls then flatten slightly. Grill on BBQ or George Forman Grill.

- 2 to 3 Large Romaine Lettuce Leaves

- 1/2 Italian Tomato Sliced

- 1/4 Thick Onion Slice

- Mustard (Zero Calorie)

- Ketchup (see recipe)

  I cut the turkey burger in half then lay on one leaf of romaine. Add your tomato, onion mustard and ketchup. Cover with other leaf, like a long hamburger bun :)Serve with Cucumber Salad or Green Salad.

# Hamburger

- 3.95 oz of 95% Lean Hamburger

- 1 tsp. Onion Powder

- 1 tsp. Garlic Powder

- 1 tbsp Cumin

- 1 tsp. Cayenne Pepper (Optional)

- 1 tsp. Paprika

- 1 Clove of Garlic

- Salt and Pepper to taste

    <u>Directions:</u> Roll hamburger into balls then flatten slightly. Grill on BBQ or George Forman Grill.

- 2 to 3 Large Romaine Lettuce Leaves

- 1/2 Italian Tomato Sliced

- 1/4 Thick Onion Slice

- Mustard (Zero Calorie)

- Ketchup (see recipe)

    <u>Directions:</u> I cut the hamburger burger in half then lay on one leaf of romaine. Add your tomato, onion mustard and ketchup. Cover with other leaf, like a long hamburger bun :) Serve with Cucumber Salad or Green Salad.

# DESSERTS

# Phase III

## Chocolate Pudding

- 10 oz. Soft Tofu

- 1/2 C Cocoa

- 1/2 to 3/4 Banana

- 4-6 package of Vanilla Stevia 4-6 to taste

- 1/2 C Soy Milk

- Vanilla to taste

> Directions: Mix together in a food possessor (adding any ingredient to taste) Refrigerate 8 to 12 hours 1 Tablespoon 62 calories

## Chocolate, Peanut Butter Pudding

- ⮕ 19 oz. Soft Tofu

- ⮕ 1/4 C Cocoa

- ⮕ 1 tbsp. Peanut Butter

- ⮕ 2/3 to 1 Banana

- ⮕ 4 packets of Vanilla Stevia

- ⮕ Vanilla to taste

Directions: Mix together in a food possessor (adding any ingredient to taste) Refrigerate 8 to 12 hours.

*Calories: 1/2 Cup approximately 98*

# Carob Walnut Cookies

- 4 to 6 Medjool Dates (Pitted) or 1 C. Raisins

- 3/4 C raw walnuts

- 1/4 C raw carob powder

- 1/8 tsp. sea salt

- Vanilla to taste

Directions: Combine the dates (or raisins), walnuts, carob powder, salt and vanilla in the food processor. Process until the dough begins sticking together.

Press the dough into 2-inch cookie cutters placed on a sheet tray lined with parchment paper. Shoot for a thickness of 1/3- to 1/2-inch. Or, make 1- to 1 1/2-inch balls and flatten.

Place the cookies in the freezer to chill and firm up for 30 minutes or more before serving or transferring to the fridge for serving later.

Will keep for many weeks in the fridge or freezer. Thaw 5 minutes before eating.

*I also form the cookies into a small bowl (press together in a ball and press your finger in the middle to create a bowl) then fill with 1/2 t peanut butter. YUMMMM!

*Calories: 98 (12 cookies)*

## Chocolate Bar

- 1/2 C Coconut Oil

- 1/2 C Cacao Powder

- 1/4 C Maple syrup

- 2 package Vanilla Stevia

- 1 tsp. Vanilla extract

- 1/2 C Chopped or Whole Almonds

Directions: Blend liquid ingredients until super smooth. You can add more sweeteners or more chocolate to suit your tastes. Transfer mixture to separate bowl and stir in almonds. (Feel free to add other goodies...coconut, berries, etc). Spread on a plastic wrap lined plate or dish and place in freezer to cool.

Calories: 39 per piece (35 pieces)

# Chocolate Peanut Butter Cups

- 1/2 C Coconut Oil

- 1/2 C Cacao Powder

- 1/4 C Maple syrup

- 2 packets Vanilla Stevia

- 1 tsp. Vanilla extract

- *Peanut butter amount will vary

- *Plastic Egg Tray

Directions: Blend liquid ingredients until super smooth. You can add more sweetener or more chocolate to suit your tastes. Line each egg slot with plastic wrap. Fill each slot with 1 teaspoon of chocolate. Immediately place 1 teaspoon of peanut butter on chocolate. If you wish pour more chocolate on peanut butter, then place in freezer for 15 to 30 minutes.

* I would fill one egg holder at a time with chocolate and peanut butter to ensure a complete peanut butter cup.

Calories: 121 per cup (12 cups)

# Lemon Pudding

- 10 oz. Soft Tofu

- Lemon Juice  2 to 3 lemons

- Lemon Zest - 1 1/2 lemons

- 1 Lime - Juice and zest

- 10 oz. Soft Tofu

- 4 package Vanilla Stevia

- 1 Banana

- Vanilla to taste

Directions: Mix together in a food processor (adding or taking away any ingredient to taste)
Optional: Blueberries on top if desire

*Calories: 176 (1/2 cup)*

# Crust

- 1/2 C Almonds

- 1/2 C Walnuts

- 6 to 9 Medjool Dates

- 1/4 to 1/2 C Shredded Coconut

- 1 tsp. Vanilla

Directions: Combine nuts in food processor. Add dates (no seed) coconut and vanilla.

Press in a 9x13 baking dish. Place in the freezer for 20 minutes minimum. (You can add more of any ingredient depending on the texture you desire. Also any nut may be used. Preferable one hard nut ex. macadamia and or one soft nut ex. pecan)

*Calories:* 103 (12 servings)

# Fruit Tart

- ⮑ 1 C. Peanut Butter

- ⮑ 2 1/2 Bananas (sliced)

- ⮑ 1 C Blueberry's

- ⮑ 2 C Strawberry's (quarter sliced)

- ⮑ 2 packets Stevia

- ⮑ 1 Nut Crust (See Recipe)

Directions: Prepare your crust. After crust has set in freezer for 20 minutes or more spread peanut butter on top. Slice bananas and layer on top of peanut butter. Combine blueberry, strawberry and stevia in a bowl and combine. Layer fruit mixture on top of bananas. Refrigerate for an hour and enjoy. * You can use any fruit mixture you like.

*Approximately 317 calories per square (12 squares)*

## Lemon Tart

- Nut Crust (See Recipe)

- Lemon Pudding (See Recipe)

- 1/4 C Blueberry's (Decoration on top)

  <u>Directions:</u> Prepare Crust and place 1/4 Cup in custard or tart dishes. Freeze for 20 minutes, minimum. Spoon lemon pudding in prepared dishes. Top with blueberries.

  *Approximately 276 Calories per dish*

# Chocolate, Peanut Butter, Banana Tart

⊃ Nut Crust (See Recipe)

⊃ 1/2 C Peanut Butter (sliced)

⊃ 2 Bananas

⊃ Chocolate, Peanut Butter, Banana Pudding (See Recipe)

⊃ Cocoa Nips

Directions: Prepare Crust and place 1/4 Cup in custard or tart dishes. Freeze for 20 minutes, minimum. Spread 1 Tablespoon of peanut butter on top of crust in each tart dish. Layer sliced bananas on top of peanut butter. Spoon chocolate and peanut butter pudding on bananas, sprinkle cocoa nips for decoration.

*Calories:* 125 a piece (12 pieces)

# Chocolate, Peanut Butter Mousse

⮕ Chocolate, Peanut Butter Pudding (Recipe)

⮕ 1/2 C. Greek Yogurt (or to taste)

<u>Directions:</u> Combine chocolate, peanut butter pudding with Greek yogurt. Calories 52 1/2 C

# Jayne's Birthday Cake

(Not a cake it's a pie) aka **Chocolate Peanut butter Mouse Pie**

## Crust

- ⮑ 1/2 C Almonds

- ⮑ 1/2 C Walnuts

- ⮑ 6 to 9 Medjool Dates

- ⮑ 1/4 to 1/2 C Shredded Coconut

- ⮑ 1 t Vanilla

    <u>Directions:</u> Combine nuts in processor. Add dates (no seed) coconut and vanilla.
    Press in a 9x13 baking dish. Place in the freezer for 20 minutes minimum.

    (You can add more of any ingredient depending on the texture you desire. Also any nut may be used. Preferable one hard nut ex. macadamia and or one soft nut ex. pecan)

    <u>*Calories:*</u> *125 a piece (12 pieces)*

## 1st Layer

- Chocolate
- 1/2 C Coconut Oil
- 1/2 C Cacao Powder
- 1/4 C Maple Syrup
- 2 packets Vanilla Stevia
- 1 t Vanilla Extract

Blend liquid ingredients until super smooth. You can add more sweeteners or more chocolate to suit your tastes. Pour onto crust. Place in the freezer for 15 minutes or until chocolate is hard.

## 2nd Layer

- Peanut Butter

Spread Peanut Butter on top of chocolate. Place in freezer for 15 minutes.

## 3rd Layer

- Chocolate Pudding
- 10 oz. Soft Tofu
- 1/2 C Cocoa
- 1/2 to 1 Banana
- 4-6 pkts of Vanilla Stevia 4-6 to taste
- 1/2 C Soy Milk
- Vanilla to taste

Mix together in a food possessor (adding any ingredient to taste). Pour pudding on top of peanut butter. Place in the freezer for 15 to 30 minutes then transfer into the refrigerator.

*Calories: 636 per serving (6 servings)*

# Flour-less Peanut Butter Cookies

- 1 cup smooth peanut butter
- 1 cup Stevia
- 2 whole egg
- 1 tsp baking soda
- 1 tsp vanilla

Directions: In a medium bowl with a wooden spoon, beat peanut butter until it becomes slightly creamier. Add sugar and mix well. Finally, add the whole egg and mix.

When well blended, drop by spoonfuls onto a greased cookie sheet or spray with cooking spray to prevent from sticking. Bake at 350°F degrees for about 12-15 minutes or until you see them golden brown at the bottom; makes about 12 to 19 cookies. You can double the recipe.

*Calories: 92 per cookie*

## Disclaimer

The Recipes in The HCG Body for Life Recipe Book – Phase III are only for people that are currently moving into Phase III or in Phase III (Maintenance) or simply just want to use these recipes to maintain a healthier diet or lifestyle.